Stephen Arterburn
Kenny Luck with Mike Yorkey

every young man,
God's man
workbook

Pursuing Confidence, Courage, and Commitment

D1399984

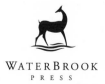

WATERBROOK
PRESS

EVERY YOUNG MAN, GOD'S MAN WORKBOOK
PUBLISHED BY WATERBROOK PRESS
2375 Telstar Drive, Suite 160
Colorado Springs, Colorado 80920
A division of Random House, Inc.

Quotations from *Every Young Man, God's Man* © 2005 by Kenny Luck and Stephen Arterburn.

All Scripture quotations, unless otherwise indicated, are taken from the *Holy Bible, New International Version*®. NIV®. Copyright © 1973, 1978, 1984 by International Bible Society. Used by permission of Zondervan Publishing House. All rights reserved. Scripture quotations marked (MSG) are taken from *The Message*. Copyright © 1993, 1994, 1995, 1996, 2000, 2001, 2002. Used by permission of NavPress Publishing Group.

Italics in Scripture quotations reflect the authors' added emphasis.

Details in some anecdotes and stories have been changed to protect the identities of the persons involved.

ISBN 1-57856-984-2

Printed in the United States of America
2005—First Edition

10 9 8 7 6 5 4 3 2 1

What Readers Are Saying About
Every Young Man, God's Man
by Stephen Arterburn and Kenny Luck with Mike Yorkey

"Every Young Man, God's Man pulls no punches in challenging young men to declare their loyalty to Jesus Christ early and not waver in a lifelong pursuit of His ways and plans. All important issues are explored with refreshing candor—from personal holiness to sexual purity to spiritual warfare and more. Every young man eager to make his life count will gain huge benefits from this book."

—JOSH MCDOWELL, author and speaker

"Every Young Man, God's Man does more than just warn young men of the dangers that lurk in the shadows of adolescence. It gives them hope that they can overcome and conquer their fears. Every chapter is filled with the kind of practical, down-to-earth advice that will arm young men against the assaults of sexual temptation, peer pressure, and isolation.… No overly simplistic solutions found here; just solid scriptural principles that create godly young men. My sons will read this book—very soon!"

—ROSS PARSLEY, associate pastor of New Life Church

"Kenny Luck has a brave and raw style that grabs you by the throat and, at the same time, gently moves you to want to change. He is able to talk about the dark, secret, and tough places that most guys would prefer to keep secret. He says things that others only think of saying with the clear intent to help guys experience God's love and power for their lives."

—DOUG FIELDS, pastor to students at Saddleback Church,
author, speaker, and president of Simply Youth Ministry

contents

questions you may have about this workbook

What will the *Every Young Man, God's Man Workbook* do for me?

Are you making progress where it counts? Are you dealing with the same character issues or fighting the same battles you fought a year ago? Are your relationships improving? Are you closing the gap between what you believe and how you really live? Many young Christian men are discouraged by their honest answers to these questions. But there is hope: God has a plan to help His young men complete the personal drive toward spiritual maturity and genuine manhood.

Part of the acclaimed Every Man series by popular counselor and speaker Stephen Arterburn, this workbook is specially designed to help you personalize and apply the groundbreaking principles revealed in the best-selling book, *Every Young Man, God's Man*. Participants will be encouraged to evaluate where they are in their spiritual journeys; to become more intimate with God and truly give Him every area of their lives; and to live lives of lasting quality, purpose, and integrity.

Is this workbook enough or do I also need the book *Every Young Man, God's Man*?

Included in each weekly study you'll find a number of excerpts from the book *Every Young Man, God's Man,* each one marked at the beginning and end by this symbol: 📖 Nevertheless, your best approach is to also read the book *Every Young Man, God's Man* as you go through this companion workbook. You'll find the appropriate chapters listed at the beginning of each weekly study.

The lessons look long. Do I need to work through each one?

This workbook is designed to promote your thorough exploration of all the material, but you may find it best to focus your time and discussion on some sections and questions more than others.

To help your pacing, we've designed the workbook so it can most easily be used in either an eight-week or twelve-week approach.

- For the eight-week track, simply follow along with the basic organization already set up with the eight different weekly lessons.
- For the twelve-week track, the lessons marked for Weeks 2, 5, 6, and 7 as shown can be divided into two parts (you'll see the dividing place marked in the text).

(In addition, of course, you may decide to follow at an even slower pace, whether you're going through the workbook individually or in a group.)

Above all, keep in mind that the purpose of the workbook is to help guide you in specific life application of the biblical truths taught in *Every Young Man, God's Man.* The wide range of questions included in each weekly study is meant to help you approach this practical application from different angles and with personal reflection and self-examination. Allowing adequate time to prayerfully reflect on each question will be much more valuable to you than rushing through this workbook.

in the man zone
or just a poser?

This week's reading assignment:

chapters 1–2 in *Every Young Man, God's Man*

At one time, I was stupid enough to believe that I could play Christian and also play cool with the party and girl scene at school. I'll never forget one hottie telling me, "You are like the perfect blend of religious and cool."…

[But] you're in the Man Zone now. The game has changed. Old ways don't cut it anymore.

—from chapter 1 in *Every Young Man, God's Man*

EVERY YOUNG MAN'S TRUTH
(Your Personal Journey into God's Word)

As you begin this first study, take some time to check out the Bible passages below. They'll tell you about integrity, loyalty, and being the real you, no matter what people think. In fact, the three men in these scriptures are great mentors for you as you strive to become God's young man. King

David learned to accept testing from God as a way to grow stronger. General Joshua drew a line in the sand and declared, "I'm for God. Period." And Jesus, even in His human nature, refused to let peoples' opinions get Him off track. He had a mission to accomplish, and He stuck to it. These men lead the way into the Man Zone. Are you willing to follow?

David praised the LORD in the presence of the whole assembly, saying, "Praise be to you, O LORD, God of our father Israel, from everlasting to everlasting....

"I know, my God, that you test the heart and are pleased with integrity. All these things have I given willingly and with honest intent. And now I have seen with joy how willingly your people who are here have given to you." (1 Chronicles 29:10,17)

Joshua said to all the people: "This is what the LORD, the God of Israel, says: 'Long ago your forefathers, including Terah the father of Abraham and Nahor, lived beyond the River and worshiped other gods. But I took your father Abraham from the land beyond the River and led him throughout Canaan and gave him many descendants. I gave him Isaac, and to Isaac I gave Jacob and Esau. I assigned the hill country of Seir to Esau, but Jacob and his sons went down to Egypt.

"'Then I sent Moses and Aaron, and I afflicted the Egyptians by what I did there, and I brought you out. When I brought your fathers out of Egypt, you came to the sea, and the Egyptians pursued them with chariots and horsemen as far as the Red Sea....'

"Now fear the LORD and serve him with all faithfulness. Throw away the gods your forefathers worshiped beyond the River and in Egypt, and serve the LORD. But if serving the LORD seems undesirable to you, then choose for yourselves this day whom you will serve.… But as for me and my household, we will serve the LORD." (Joshua 24:2-6,14-15)

They came to him and said, "Teacher, we know you are a man of integrity. You aren't swayed by men, because you pay no attention to who they are; but you teach the way of God in accordance with the truth. Is it right to pay taxes to Caesar or not?" (Mark 12:14)

1. King David knew that God tests our hearts. What good—or joy— can come from this? How have you seen this work in your own life?

2. Joshua was an army general who had to keep his loyalties straight amid constant battles. Remembering God's great works of the past helped him do it. So list some of the ways God has worked in your own life so far. How does this make you feel?

3. Even Jesus' enemies considered Him a man of integrity. According to them, how did Jesus show this integrity? When is it toughest for you to "pay no attention" to what others think of you?

4. Think about the most recent situation when this question was a big deal for you: Where is your loyalty going to lie? What did you do?

☑ EVERY YOUNG MAN'S CHOICE
(Questions for Personal Reflection and Examination)

📖 You're becoming a man, and that means you have to start thinking like one. Similarly, to become God's man, you have to think like one of His sons. To help you think like God's man, you need to think through the following statements that I've come up with. I call them "Kenny's Code." Read each one slowly.

📖 Before you get into tough situations as a man, you have to get your identity settled and strong. Then you can focus on being who you are versus someone who oscillates between God Guy and Poser Guy, between Sunday Guy and Tequila Shooter Guy, or between Bible Study Man and Porn Studies Man. 📖

5. Go back and review the statements in Kenny's Code. Think: Which of these do I already believe? Which of them do I need to believe?

6. Think about someone who knows of you just by seeing you around. If this person were asked *what defines your identity*, what do you think he or she would say? Why? (What about a guy you hang out with all the time?)

7. Recall the story of Jim, the guy who was a poser during his high-school years. Which of his faces do you tend to wear during a routine day? What would it take for you to start wearing your real face more often?

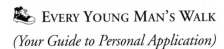 EVERY YOUNG MAN'S WALK
(Your Guide to Personal Application)

📖 One night I would hang out with my Christian friends at a Bible study, and the next night I would be laughing my head off at a huge beer bash with the "stoners." It's a good thing that I had friends praying that God would rattle my world and get me back on track. I needed my cage rattled, because there were parts of me that really liked the feelings of acceptance and the danger of dancing with sin. What I didn't like was the war raging within me, which made me miserable. But I never discussed those feelings with anyone. 📖

📖 So many men, young and old, are caught between competing identities that divide their loyalty, just like Brandon. Maybe you've worn a mask or rationalized your faith away when it's been uncomfortable. If your inner loyalty and commitment to Christ is divided, how can you expect to overcome the fear of what other people think about your being a Christian? Moving into the Man Zone means… having a clear and personal picture of Jesus Christ's passion for you on the cross and then letting your heart match His with love and loyalty. 📖

8. Kenny talks about nights with the Bible and nights with the stoners. Can you see any splits like this in your own actions? What kind of world rattling could help you?

9. Suppose you feel your loyalty is divided. Do you agree with Kenny that "having a clear and personal picture of Jesus Christ's passion for you" will meet your need? Why?

10. When could you spend some quiet time prayerfully remembering how much Jesus loves you? Jot your weekly schedule below and make your plans.

11. Kenny says: "I am in your space to remind you that your loyalty will be tested so that your spiritual backbone can develop." On a scale of 1 to 5, how strong is your backbone at the moment? What prayer would you like to lift to God about this right now?

12. In quietness, review what you have written and learned in this week's study. If further thoughts or prayer requests come to your mind and heart, you may want to write them here.

13. What for you was the most meaningful concept or truth in this week's study?

How would you talk this over with God? Write your response here as a prayer to Him.

What do you believe God wants you to do in response to this week's study?

👤👤 Every Young Man's Talk

(Constructive Topics and Questions for Group Discussion)

Key Highlights from the Book for Reading Aloud and Discussing

📖 For the first time in my life, I expressed to God what I really wanted more than anything—a real encounter with Him.… He knew I had been deliberately fooling myself, but He also saw someone who was experiencing turmoil regarding who Christ was. When I expressed a longing from deep within my heart—as simple as it was—He seized that measly effort to invade my room and bring me closer to Him as never before. 📖

📖 God had told Hezekiah that he was going to die, which would certainly get my attention. In response, Hezekiah dialed 911, and amazingly, he was granted a fifteen-year extension on earth! While Hezekiah knew God was all-powerful, he also knew that God was also a *rewarder* of those loyal to him, and that a "loyal heart" produced "what was good in Your sight." 📖

📖 I was enrolling at UCLA, that bastion of babes, beer, and beach time.… We're talking Babeville with the hottest-looking girls on your left, on your right, and dead ahead, but I was committed to honoring God and remaining loyal to Him. I made that commitment public; I let other people in on the fact that I was a Christian. 📖

Discussion Questions

An opening question: Which parts of these chapters were most helpful or encouraging to you? Why?

A. What do you *really* want more than anything? How can you tell?

B. Review the story of Hezekiah in 2 Kings 20:1-6. What does this story tell you about a loyal heart? If you were to do a quick heart check right now, what would be your L.Q. (Loyalty Quotient)?

C. Have you ever lived in—or visited—Babeville? Was that cool for you? How hard or easy is it for you to go public with your Christian identity in that town? Talk it over!

D. Together, review the closing paragraphs of chapter 1 in the book, which tell what you'll be learning in the coming chapters. Share about which one or two topics you most want to explore.

E. Kenny talks about admiring guys who work hard on their sport or craft in order to be successful. But we don't get it when it comes to training to become God's young men. What kinds of practical training brings this kind of success? (Tell about what has helped you the most.)

F. To close out this first session, ask one of the guys to read aloud Proverbs 10:9 and 11:3. Discuss what's so great about walking in integrity—and then pray for one another's walk during the coming week.

hard to do:
no mind games!

This week's reading assignment:

chapters 3–4 in *Every Young Man, God's Man*

"When I am alone with my temptations, I choose pleasure. Feeling like I'm all alone in it makes the situation worse and causes me to be spiritually lazy. On the other hand, when I am with friends or can interrupt the temptation with a phone call, prayer, exercise, or something else, then that interruption keeps me out of the situation."…

Here's my point: you are not alone when you admit your battle with sexual temptation, and you are not alone if you fail.

—from chapter 3 in *Every Young Man, God's Man*

📖 EVERY YOUNG MAN'S TRUTH
(Your Personal Journey into God's Word)

What's your most treasured reward for good work, a nice performance, a fine sports season? You've probably got those trophies and ribbons sitting on a shelf somewhere, right? But what about rewards in your life with God? Here, too, you can win awesome payoffs. Because *God rewards obedience.* The scriptures below will help you understand the reward for embracing and acting upon the truth. And they'll encourage you to stay disciplined in your efforts against temptation.

It's true that you're saved only by God's grace and could never earn His favor. But that doesn't mean you can't please Him by following His will. When you choose His ways, He loves to give you the high-five.

Do not store up for yourselves treasures on earth, where moth and rust destroy, and where thieves break in and steal. But store up for yourselves treasures in heaven. (Matthew 6:19-20)

So we make it our goal to please him, whether we are at home in the body or away from it. For we must all appear before the judgment seat of Christ, that each one may receive what is due him for the things done while in the body, whether good or bad. (2 Corinthians 5:9-10)

Consider him who endured such opposition from sinful men, so that you will not grow weary and lose heart.

In your struggle against sin, you have not yet resisted to the point of shedding your blood. And you have forgotten that word of encouragement that addresses you as sons:

"My son, do not make light of the Lord's discipline,
   and do not lose heart when he rebukes you,
because the Lord disciplines those he loves,
   and he punishes everyone he accepts as a son."

Endure hardship as discipline; God is treating you as sons. For what son is not disciplined by his father? If you are not disciplined (and everyone undergoes discipline), then you are illegitimate children and not true sons. Moreover, we have all had human fathers who disciplined us and we respected them for it. How much more should we submit to the Father of our spirits and live! Our fathers disciplined us for a little while as they thought best; but God disciplines us for our good, that we may share in his holiness. No discipline seems pleasant at the time, but painful. Later on, however, it produces a harvest of righteousness and peace for those who have been trained by it. (Hebrews 12:3-11)

1. What is the difference between storing up treasures on earth and in heaven? Where is your biggest bank account located at the moment?

2. On the cross Jesus suffered the full penalty and judgment for our sins. While we won't be judged, the quality of our works on earth will be judged some day. How does this make you feel?

3. How is Jesus a great example of sticking with obedience, no matter what?

4. What are some of the rewards of accepting God's discipline, according to the author of Hebrews?

Section I: focus on chapter 3. Note: for an eight-week study, include Section II starting on page 22.

☑ EVERY YOUNG MAN'S CHOICE
(Questions for Personal Reflection and Examination)

📖 I recently asked a room of young men, ages seventeen to twenty-one, to take an anonymous survey that contained the following question: what are the top three battles you face as a younger man?

One hundred percent of them—every guy in the room—wrote that sexual temptation, lust, masturbation, or porn topped his list. 📖

📖 I believe that being a Christian and having character are not the same thing. When God entered your life, you instantly inherited many things. You were forgiven of all your sins, you became a child of God, and you were placed spiritually in heaven with Christ.…

[But] a fundamental change in your character traits (who you are and how you react under pressure) was *not* on the list. God has chosen to bring us character only when we decide to do hard things that require faith in His way. 📖

5. Why is sexual temptation so high on the list of battles for most guys? Of the listed reasons why guys *lose* this battle, which most closely relates to your own struggles?

6. God made character development a growth process. In your opinion, why didn't He just give you a good character when He made you His child?

👟 EVERY YOUNG MAN'S WALK
(Your Guide to Personal Application)

📖 Mark, for example, knew exactly what God's plan for sex was, but he rationalized and debated with himself about the whole idea of remaining pure. Once the debate began in his mind, he worked through various scenarios regarding his girlfriend, Kelly. Like a kitchen faucet with a slow leak under the cabinet, Mark began allowing certain things to happen. For instance, their good-bye kiss went from a peck to a full-on session of deep kissing. He figured that was okay because everyone still had their clothes on. 📖

📖 When you resist change, however, God has other ways to get our character in order, and those usually involve His calling a time-out on your plans. God can forge character by allowing difficulties, delays, or even the consequences of your choices to act as His agents of change. The Bible is filled with examples of His making men uncomfortable so He could teach them something about character. Just ask these guys: Joseph…Moses…David…Jonah…Job…Paul. 📖

7. Recall the story of Mark and Kelly. If you were Mark's best friend, what advice would you have given him at the beginning of his relationship with Kelly?

8. When has God made you uncomfortable in order to get you to change? Of the six biblical characters listed, which has the most to teach you, personally, about this? Why?

9. Kenny says that "God's young man risks letting God be in control and managing him freely." But what's the big risk? What is the scariest part for you?

10. What for you was the most meaningful concept or truth in chapter 3 of *Every Young Man, God's Man?*

    How would you talk this over with God? Write your response here as a prayer to Him.

    What do you believe God wants you to do in response to this week's study?

🔲🔲 EVERY YOUNG MAN'S TALK
(Constructive Topics and Questions for Group Discussion)

Key Highlights from the Book for Reading Aloud and Discussing

📖 God's men have a long-range plan. God's men think through questions—tough questions. Have you ever asked yourself:

- Why can't I grow past sexual temptations and thoughts?
- Why am I not getting closer to the standard I know is right?
- Why do I keep repeating the same mistakes over and over?

If you are asking yourself these questions, then you are searching for the one thing that separates the men from the boys—character. 📖

📖 God's man Hosea was speaking to a group of spiritually immature men in Israel. He used their knowledge of farming to explain God's work in their lives and how they could be productive for him. The picture he painted was the all-too-familiar one about hard work and sweat paying off at harvest time. Any good Israelite knew that a fruitful yield started with the condition of the soil. Hard soil was bad, and soft soil was good. Hard soil offered little chance of taking the seed, while tilled land yielded a crop—perhaps a bountiful one. The farmer had to do the hard work (breaking up the unplowed ground) to get the results.

Hosea's metaphor works today as well. If you want to be God's man on the outside, you've got to pull out the jackhammer and get to work on the inside. 📖

📖 One of the most difficult things I have ever done was to talk about this [masturbation] habit with the men in my Bible study. It was also one of the best things I ever did. When I confessed my situation to my brothers, God gave me the strength to say no to the flesh and say yes to His Spirit in the moments of testing. He knew it took guts for me to give up my "dirty little secret." He knew it required faith and humility because I risked rejection for a stronger walk with God. 📖

Discussion Questions

An opening question: Which parts of this chapter were most helpful or encouraging to you? Why?

A. Are you a boy or a man (based on the questions you ask yourself)?

B. What would it mean for you to pull out the jackhammer and work on your inside? Be as specific as possible.

C. Why is it so hard to talk about our dirty little secrets with other guys who care about us? What helps you gain the courage to do it?

D. Kenny says: "You can't necessarily expect immediate results when you choose to do the right thing." In your experience, what can you expect?

E. How do you react when you hear God saying no to you?

F. Kenny makes this statement: "Sometimes God's will *feels* like a cruel joke—even sucks, if you're honest." Tell about a time when this was true for you. How did you deal with it?

Section II: focus on chapter 4.

Note: if you're following a twelve-week track,
save the rest of this lesson for the following week.
If you're on the eight-week track…then keep going.

☑ EVERY YOUNG MAN'S CHOICE
(Questions for Personal Reflection and Examination)

📖 My appetite for pleasure and fun controlled my life. Why should I say no to what I wanted to do? I was young enough, insecure enough, and lonely enough *not* to listen to the voice in my head questioning some of my decisions. While I am ashamed to reveal everything about my BC (before Christ) days, they reveal a fundamental truth about me: when it was in my interest, I was a pro at playing mind games to get what I wanted when I wanted it. 📖

📖 Our actions reveal our true heart and our maturity in Christ. When Jesus shows up on your porch with some truth about your present direction, an attitude that needs adjustment, or an action that needs to be addressed, how do you react? 📖

11. What are some of your favorite mind games for getting what you want?

12. In the second quotation above, how do you answer Kenny's question about your reaction to Jesus?

EVERY YOUNG MAN'S WALK
(Your Guide to Personal Application)

📖 Danny used these same mind games when he complained to Ashley that she didn't really love him. When they started dating four months earlier, he respected her virginity. He bought into the "true love waits" motto. But as he daily fantasized about her, the whole virginity thing became less attractive to him. He resented the firewall she had installed regarding physical intimacy.

Danny's mind became one track—and it was no longer on God. 📖

📖 His parents were right, but Tom could not admit that. He fought them tooth and nail about getting a summer job to pay for *his* car insurance, *his* gas, and *his* car repairs. His mom and dad told him that since he was not taking summer school classes, the next three months would be a great time to find a part-time job to cover his car-related expenses.…

He had other things on his mind—like sleeping in and hanging out with his friends. 📖

13. How could Danny change so much in just four months? If you were Danny, what could you have done to help yourself stick with "true love waits"?

14. Have you ever been like Tom? What did he learn about a man's responsibility—and what have *you* learned so far?

15. Carefully read John 4:4-30, focusing on verse 23. Think: how would you answer Kenny's five questions about self-honesty?

   a. Am I being honest with myself about my spiritual commitment to Christ?

   b. Am I being totally honest with God about my life?

c. Have I been honest with others about my spiritual life and struggles?

d. Am I willing to hear the truth from God and other brothers about my spiritual direction?

e. Will I do what they say?

16. What for you was the most meaningful concept or truth in chapter 4 of *Every Young Man, God's Man?*

How would you talk this over with God? Write your response here as a prayer to Him.

What do you believe God wants you to do in response to this week's study?

☺☺ EVERY YOUNG MAN'S TALK

(Constructive Topics and Questions for Group Discussion)

Key Highlights from the Book for Reading Aloud and Discussing

📖 I bet you've rationalized a few things. You wouldn't be normal if you haven't. It's easy to do. All you have to do is repeat one of the following excuses… 📖

📖 All of us will stand before God one day and have to account for our actions today. You want that day to be a great one. He won't accept your bogus excuses for why you traded in your commitment to Him for cheap physical thrills or moments of gratification. What will you say to the Lord—the same Lord who reads all your thoughts and exposes your mind games? That's why, when facing a moral dilemma, you have one of two ways to go: either face up to the truth or run from God. 📖

📖 The best habit you can get into is seeing how God's purposes for bringing truth to your life are all about *you!* He's doing this because he loves you. He may be telling you things you may not *want* to hear, but they are things that you *need* to hear to become God's young man. The fact is that He can't help Himself—He *is* the truth. So how do you know when God's speaking His truth to you? It's God talking when… 📖

Discussion Questions

An opening question: Which parts of this chapter were most helpful or encouraging to you? Why?

G. Read the first quotation above, then check out the excuses that Kenny lists in the book on pages 45-46. Talk about which of these you've used at one time or another. What were the results?

H. Do you agree that facing a moral dilemma offers you only two choices? Can you share a personal example about this?

I. In the past, what things has God told you that you didn't want to hear? (What is He telling you right now?)

J. Kenny says: "Sometimes accepting the truth is hard because *change requires action*, which can produce tension." Where do you feel the tension when you face a tough truth about yourself?

K. God sometimes acts like a surgeon with us, cutting in order to heal us. Are you down with going under the knife? Talk it over.

L. Kenny states that God will eventually out us to get our attention. What does he mean?

M. How would you like to pray for one another before closing your group time?

knowing better than to blend

This week's reading assignment:

chapters 5–6 in *Every Young Man, God's Man*

Our whole mission was to let loose, have fun, and play around. That's why all of us bought into every experience the world had to offer. But when we became high-school seniors, we were getting tired of the party and girl scene. It was just stale. In fact, I remember tape-recording a late-night conversation at my kitchen table with some of the guys. Out of the blue I asked my friend Pat, "What would you do if Jesus Christ were here right now?"

—from chapter 6 in *Every Young Man, God's Man*

EVERY YOUNG MAN'S TRUTH
(Your Personal Journey into God's Word)

You live in the world. But how much of the world lives in you? Can you be God's young man and blend perfectly with the culture too? According to the scriptures below, it's impossible. Check them out. As you do, ask yourself what it means, in practical terms, that Christ has called you *out* of the world to be His servant *in* the world: What do you watch? What do you listen to? Who do you hang out with?

Yes, you need to have non-Christian friends if you are to be a witness. You need to understand the values and priorities of others if you are to influence them for Christ. But be wise in the way you go about it. Don't let the world form you into it's mold. Know better than to blend.

> If the world hates you, keep in mind that it hated me first. If you belonged to the world, it would love you as its own. As it is, you do not belong to the world, but I have chosen you out of the world. That is why the world hates you. (John 15:18-19)

> You adulterous people, don't you know that friendship with the world is hatred toward God? Anyone who chooses to be a friend of the world becomes an enemy of God. Or do you think Scripture says without reason that the spirit he caused to live in us tends toward envy, but he gives us more grace? That is why Scripture says:

> "God opposes the proud
> but gives grace to the humble."

> Submit yourselves, then, to God. Resist the devil, and he will flee from you. Come near to God and he will come near to you. Wash your hands, you sinners, and purify your hearts, you double-minded. Grieve, mourn and wail. Change your laughter to mourning and your joy to gloom. Humble yourselves before the Lord, and he will lift you up. (James 4:4-10)

> Do not love the world or anything in the world. If anyone loves the world, the love of the Father is not in him. For everything in the

world—the cravings of sinful man, the lust of his eyes and the boasting of what he has and does—comes not from the Father but from the world. The world and its desires pass away, but the man who does the will of God lives forever. (1 John 2:15-17)

1. What evidence of the world's values do you see around you? How tempting are these values for you?

2. According to James, what is the cure for being double-minded?

3. How can you tell when you are loving the world? What do you do about it?

4. What encouraging truth comes through to you in 1 John 2:15-17?

☑ EVERY YOUNG MAN'S CHOICE
(Questions for Personal Reflection and Examination)

📖 Then it happened. My car—actually, my mom's—kissed a rail-road tie. While it was just a "touch," I ended up denting the driver's side door. Now I was in deep linguine.

My first impulse was practical—save my own skin! 📖

📖 A true God's young man must abandon the middle ground and determine, in his own mind, that he cannot peacefully coexist with his enemies. This pattern of taking a strong stance is well illustrated in the Bible for us to clearly see. Think about: Moses…David… King Hezekiah…Elijah…Daniel…Jesus…Peter and John…and the believers in Revelation who were not afraid to die. 📖

5. When was the last time you were in deep linguine? What was your first impulse? your second impulse?

Jot some notes here about how you would *like* to respond the next time you land in a sticky mess:

6. Think through the challenges faced by the men Kenny lists in the second quotation above. Which of these guys do you most respect for their stance against the world? Why?

7. Kenny says that when you wreck your life, either pride will drive you, your fear will deter you, or your faith will direct you. As you look back over your life, assign percentages to each of these three motivators—pride, fear, faith. How often have you let each take control of your responses to serious hassles?

EVERY YOUNG MAN'S WALK
(Your Guide to Personal Application)

 [Some young men] are light-years apart from God when it comes to wisdom, yet they fling their "wisdom" around like *they* spoke and created the heavens and the earth. In fact, their ignorance makes them dangerous to themselves and to others. Their mind-set and actions seem to say: "Thanks for coming along for the ride, God, but I'll take the wheel from here." They would never utter those words, of course, but their *actions* say otherwise. I can just imagine God scratching His head in amazement when people shine Him on.

📔 The world wants to define what's normal for you—and it will if you let it happen. Just flip on MTV, study the newest Abercrombie & Fitch catalog, or check out the latest run of *Bachelor*. What the world values isn't hard to pick up. The world will always emphasize feelings over commitment, a free spirit over character. 📔

8. Make a two-column list below of the things you are (1) wise about, and (2) ignorant about. Then think: *Where in my life do I need more of God's wisdom?*

9. In the second quotation above, check out the sources Kenny names as places where the world's values come through. Can you come up with some specific examples of how they emphasize feelings and a free spirit? Jot your thoughts about it:

10. Go back to the stories of Jeremy and Nate. They both figured they were missing out on something. When you feel that way, where do you go to hang out? Have you told anybody about that yet?

11. In the middle of chapter 6, Kenny talks about three specific ways you might become more a friend of the world than a follower of Christ. Under each below, jot an example from your own life of an action that demonstrates your kind of friendship.

    a. You look at God's forgiveness like a credit card advance:
      How I do this…
      or, how I avoid this…

    b. You compartmentalize your behaviors:
      How I do this…
      or, how I avoid this…

    c. You allow your feelings to dominate decision making.
      How I do this…
      or, how I avoid this…

12. In quietness, review what you have written and learned in this week's study. If further thoughts or prayer requests come to your mind and heart, you may want to write them here.

13. What for you was the most meaningful concept or truth in this week's study?

How would you talk this over with God? Write your response here as a prayer to Him.

What do you believe God wants you to do in response to this week's study?

👤👤 EVERY YOUNG MAN'S TALK

(Constructive Topics and Questions for Group Discussion)

Key Highlights from the Book for Reading Aloud and Discussing

📖 Pride says [to God]: *I know better....* Fear says: *I'll miss out....* Faith says: *You know better.* 📖

📖 If you continue to resist God, He has ways of showing you that you don't know better. That's what happened to a guy named Naaman in the Bible. He was a hotshot Syrian general who was powerful, commanding, and successful. Underneath his armor, however, his body was racked by a skin disease called leprosy. On the outside—shining armor and victory. Underneath and on the inside—sores and shame. 📖

📖 Changing into God's young man requires a change in your perspective about spiritual warfare. You can no longer dismiss it, deny it, or deflect your responsibility to engage it. Instead, you must forget the notion that you can play both sides without taking it in the shorts every now and then. In other words, you cannot *blend* God's purposes with opposing purposes and practices. Specifically, you are warned not to blend with what the Bible describes as the "world." 📖

Discussion Questions

An opening question: Which parts of these chapters were most helpful or encouraging to you? Why?

A. Which of the three voices did you listen to for most of your day yesterday—pride, fear, or faith? How could you tell?

B. Together, go back over the story of General Naaman (see 2 Kings 5:1-14). How did God teach this tough guy humility?

C. How do you define spiritual warfare? In light of Kenny's comments about it, what is your win-loss record over the past month?

D. Kenny talks about the moment in a game when a team surrenders to its fate. Have you ever reached that point with God? What could you share with the other guys about this?

E. Kenny entered UCLA "trying real hard to be cool so people would like me." How cool are you at the moment, dude? Who seems to be impressed?

F. A dead squirrel taught the author: don't delay the instinct to obey. If you agree, tell why.

G. What are your prayer requests to share with the other guys?

out of the dark into defense

This week's reading assignment:

chapters 7–8 in *Every Young Man, God's Man*

The "dark side" was made famous by the Star Wars *trilogies and epitomized by the infamous character Darth Vader. While he and the other* Star Wars *characters are thoroughly the stuff of Hollywood, the saga's core theme reflects a biblical reality, which is this: every man has a dark side, something pulling him to do the wrong thing. This force inside him wages war against his noblest intentions.*

—from chapter 7 in *Every Young Man, God's Man*

EVERY YOUNG MAN'S TRUTH
(Your Personal Journey into God's Word)

The dark side keeps pulling at you, and it's tough to say no. Even the great apostle Paul felt it as a brutal inner battle. You've been there, right? Feeling the power of temptation, wanting to do right but doing wrong instead? Then the guilt. Then the tendency to despair.

But don't give up! Scripture tells you your Lord has already won the war with sin. He calls you to live in the power of His ultimate victory. It's true that willpower can only carry you so far. At some point in your battles you must give up and let Christ carry you through. Call upon Him; as Paul knew, He is ready for the rescue.

> I realize that I don't have what it takes. I can will it, but I can't do it. I decide to do good, but I don't really do it; I decide not to do bad, but then I do it anyway. My decisions, such as they are, don't result in actions. Something has gone wrong deep within me and gets the better of me every time.
>
> It happens so regularly that it's predictable. The moment I decide to do good, sin is there to trip me up. I truly delight in God's commands, but it's pretty obvious that not all of me joins in that delight. Parts of me covertly rebel, and just when I least expect it, they take charge.
>
> I've tried everything and nothing helps. I'm at the end of my rope. Is there no one who can do anything for me? Isn't that the real question?
>
> The answer, thank God, is that Jesus Christ can and does. He acted to set things right in this life of contradictions where I want to serve God with all my heart and mind, but am pulled by the influence of sin to do something totally different. (Romans 7:18-25, MSG)

> No temptation has seized you except what is common to man. And God is faithful; he will not let you be tempted beyond what you can bear. But when you are tempted, he will also provide a way out so that you can stand up under it. (1 Corinthians 10:13)

> God's solid foundation stands firm, sealed with this inscription: "The Lord knows those who are his," and, "Everyone who confesses the name of the Lord must turn away from wickedness."

In a large house there are articles not only of gold and silver, but also of wood and clay; some are for noble purposes and some for ignoble. If a man cleanses himself from the latter, he will be an instrument for noble purposes, made holy, useful to the Master and prepared to do any good work.

Flee the evil desires of youth, and pursue righteousness, faith, love and peace, along with those who call on the Lord out of a pure heart. (2 Timothy 2:20-22)

1. The apostle Paul sometimes felt like a prisoner of the law of sin. When do you feel that way?

2. According to 1 Corinthians 10:13, what is your hope when you feel seized by temptation?

3. What does it mean for you, personally, to "flee the evil desires of youth"?

4. What is your defense plan for the next time serious temptation hits? How have you prepared your heart in advance?

☑ EVERY YOUNG MAN'S CHOICE
(Questions for Personal Reflection and Examination)

📖 This dark side phenomenon makes every man a potential double agent—capable of doing the very worst even when he desires the very best. That's why the Bible makes it clear that the enemy you *really* need to be watching out for is *you.* 📖

📖 As I work with younger men, I've seen how important it is to bottle up the Enemy at various hot gates—or what I call spiritual strongholds—so that larger battles don't have to be fought. How you defend those hot gates determines how the next ten to fifteen years will play out. The Bible warns you to position your forces "so that when the day of evil comes, you may be able to stand your ground, and after you have done everything, to stand" (Ephesians 6:13). 📖

5. Review the five "have you ever" examples of ways the dark side can make you a double agent. What is your own best example?

6. How are you positioning your forces to defend the spiritual hot gates in your life? Rate your battle position: strong or weak?

7. Take a moment to read Ephesians 6:10-18. List the armor and weapons you'll need to defend yourself against dark side attacks. Which pieces do you need to rely on more when temptation hits?

👟 EVERY YOUNG MAN'S WALK
(Your Guide to Personal Application)

📖 You may know my friend. His name is Paul—the apostle. Nearly two thousand years ago, he put into words how everyone feels when the dark side takes over our lives and our actions. Paul labeled this our "sin nature," and the previous description is found in Romans 7:18-20 (MSG). It's good to know we are in good company when it comes to this battle because we all are at war with our dark side. 📖

📖 The dark side doesn't have to influence your actions, though. You can beat him at his own game by committing to a campaign of exposing him constantly. You do that by figuring you have two types of people living in one body, and your Spirit-filled nature has to suppress the dark side—or else. 📖

8. Do you ever feel like the apostle Paul did when facing temptation? Check out Romans 7:25–8:14. How can this passage point you to the way out?

9. Kenny says that suppressing the dark side involves verbally confronting it. What verbal-confrontation phrase would work best for you. Write it here:

10. Why is the hot gate of sexual fantasizing such an important one to defend? What usually happens after your thoughts give in?

11. In quietness, review what you have written and learned in this week's study. If further thoughts or prayer requests come to your mind and heart, you may want to write them here.

12. What for you was the most meaningful concept or truth in this week's study?

How would you talk this over with God? Write your response here as a prayer to Him.

What do you believe God wants you to do in response to this week's study?

EVERY YOUNG MAN'S TALK
(Constructive Topics and Questions for Group Discussion)

Key Highlights from the Book for Reading Aloud and Discussing

In your journey with God, I know you feel the dark side lurking like a shark beneath the surface of your life. The dark side inconspicuously swims in the waters of your character, hiding in your thoughts and dropping ideas into your mind that run counter to God's plan. The dark side contradicts what constitutes sin by muddying the waters so you cannot make out the clear instruction of God's Word. Your dark side is patient until it's time to strike. 📖

📖 Josh just smiled and shook his head—letting Austin feel the stupidity of his little outburst.

"You're right," Josh replied after a long pause. "You are not me, and I am not your dad. But I am your brother—in Christ. I know you don't want to hear that right now because you can't be doing what you're doing with Jessica and still be tight with me or God. I don't care if you push me away, avoid me, or never see me again. But God can't go from being a big part of your life to a small part unless you're making space for the wrong things." 📖

📖 Each mental assault takes it toll and invests Satan with more power so that after a while temptation will *feel* irresistible. To take a cue from Kevin's story: each mental happy meal he indulged in brought the Enemy's victory closer and closer.

Hot gates must be places where you resist and make your stand—not yield. 📖

Discussion Questions

An opening question: Which parts of these chapters were most helpful or encouraging to you? Why?

A. Talk about some of the shark bites you've suffered in the past. What have you learned so far about avoiding shark-infested waters?

B. What are some of the ways Josh was being a good brother to Austin? Do you see any of these brotherly ways happening in your group? Talk it over.

C. Look at the eleven guys who yield at the hot gates (starting with Dave, Chris, and so on). For them, temptation feels irresistible. What specific brotherly advice would you give to each of these guys in their particular struggles?

D. Kenny basically says to talk to yourself when tempted. What kinds of things are you supposed to say?

E. According to Kenny: "What rocks a young guy's world is not knowing what to do when the shot clock on his temptation ticker is winding down." So what are you supposed to do as you watch that clock—and panic sets in?

F. We can't defend a hot gate without the Holy Spirit's power and direction. Review the four ways of cooperating with the Spirit (under the subhead "Defending a Hot Gate"). Then pray for one another about your areas of noncooperation!

hey Gumby: baptize that brain!

This week's reading assignment:

chapters 9–11 in *Every Young Man, God's Man*

You follow the beach master's directions to a T and meet up with your new buddies. Your new platoon leader gathers you all together to give you instructions. That's when you notice that he's holding a helmet filled with some guy's brains! His steely eyes glare at every man standing around him in a semicircle. "This is what happens to guys who don't listen to the beach master," he growls. "This whole area is mined. Go where you are told."

He didn't need to say anything more.

—from chapter 9 in *Every Young Man, God's Man*

📖 Every Young Man's Truth

(Your Personal Journey into God's Word)

What comes to mind when you think of meditating? Do you see an orange-robed monk sitting alone on a desolate hillside with closed eyes? Do you picture a new age guru lighting incense and chanting? Or do you see *yourself*—opening up the Bible and letting God's Word soak into your soul?

Stick with that third image! It is exactly what you're called to do as often as you can. Stay in the Bible; let its truths marinate your mind. Don't rush. Think it through and apply it to your everyday concerns. Really, it's pretty simple: simply delight in God's Word. You'll be blessed.

> Be strong and very courageous. Be careful to obey all the law my ser-
> vant Moses gave you; do not turn from it to the right or to the left,
> that you may be successful wherever you go. Do not let this Book of
> the Law depart from your mouth; meditate on it day and night, so
> that you may be careful to do everything written in it. Then you will
> be prosperous and successful. (Joshua 1:7-8)

> Blessed is the man
>   who does not walk in the counsel of the wicked
> or stand in the way of sinners
>   or sit in the seat of mockers.
> But his delight is in the law of the LORD,
>   and on his law he meditates day and night.
> He is like a tree planted by streams of water,
>   which yields its fruit in season
> and whose leaf does not wither.
>   Whatever he does prospers.
>   (Psalm 1:1-3)

> How can a young man keep his way pure?
>   By living according to your word.
> I seek you with all my heart;
>   do not let me stray from your commands.

I have hidden your word in my heart
that I might not sin against you.
Praise be to you, O LORD;
teach me your decrees.
With my lips I recount
all the laws that come from your mouth.
I rejoice in following your statutes
as one rejoices in great riches.
I meditate on your precepts
and consider your ways.
I delight in your decrees;
I will not neglect your word.
(Psalm 119:9-16)

1. What does being "strong and very courageous" have to do with Bible reading?

2. Do you *delight* in God's law? What other words would you use to describe your relationship to the Bible?

3. How much of God's Word have you put to memory? How does this help you stay pure?

4. Do you agree that you are what you think? If so, what does this say about the importance of meditating on Scripture?

Section I: focus on chapters 9 and 10a
(ending before the subhead "The Great Divide").
Note: for an eight-week study,
include Section II starting on page 56.

☑ EVERY YOUNG MAN'S CHOICE
(Questions for Personal Reflection and Examination)

📖 What does selective obedience look like?
- You hear what *you* want to hear.
- You reject or discount what's not in sync with *your* personal desires.
- You replace God's clear instructions with *your* own plan.
- You act out *your* plan.

Sometimes God's commands don't fit in with your "flow," your image, your friendships, or the lifestyles that go with them. So you set aside His directions because you want to be free to do what you want rather than what God wants. But just like the soldier who didn't listen to the beach master, your freedom will be short-lived.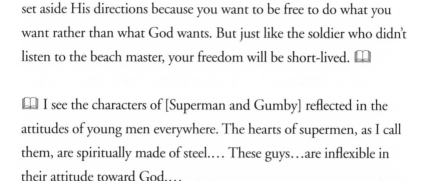

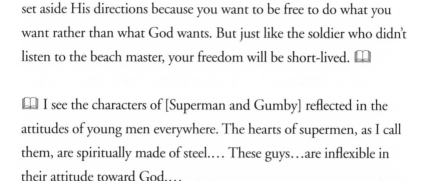 I see the characters of [Superman and Gumby] reflected in the attitudes of young men everywhere. The hearts of supermen, as I call them, are spiritually made of steel.... These guys...are inflexible in their attitude toward God....

At the other end of the spectrum are the Gumbies—guys flexible and bendable to the will of God. They might get twisted around or bent out of shape from life, but they trust the hands shaping them and their characters. They are willing to be handled like clay in the Master's hands.

5. Name some of the freedom-killing results of selective obedience that you've noticed in yourself. How is selective obedience life-destroying?

6. Are you mostly a Superman or a Gumby with God? What recent behavior gives you the best clue?

📖 EVERY YOUNG MAN'S WALK
(Your Guide to Personal Application)

📖 All men I know have felt the punishing blows that selective obedience brings. It doesn't matter who you are or what you want to become. The Bible is full of stories about great kings who could not bring themselves to complete obedience. On several occasions, good kings could not resist the impulse to fudge on God's clear instructions regarding the worship of pagan gods among His people. Allowing their subjects to build pagan shrines or "high places" among the people of God was the equivalent of erecting a statue of Osama Bin Laden in downtown Manhattan. 📖

📖 The bottom line about 80/20 guys is that their love for God is an act. They consistently put the 20 percent over their love for God. They are like the 80/20 kings of the Old Testament who allowed the high places to exist under their watch when God had said they had to go. Add it all up, and it's easy to make the argument that your 20 percent is an idol as well. 📖

7. Look at the biblical statements about three selectively obedient kings: Jehu, Joash, and Azariah. What do these scriptures tell you about God's attitude toward an "almost" complete commitment?

8. Think about your daily attitudes, words, actions, and relation-ships. Then categorize them below under: (a) the 80 percent of my life that is obedient and (b) the 20 percent of my life that is "free."

    80% Obedient   20% Free

    My insights about my 80/20 ratio are...

9. Kenny says that a humble attitude toward God is essential for the relationship to work. Study the ten benefits of a humble attitude toward God (they're printed in the book just before the subhead "The Great Divide"). Name at least three of these benefits that make you think: *It's worth it for me to humbly bow to God's will each day.*

10. What for you was the most meaningful concept or truth in chapters 9 and 10a (before the subhead "The Great Divide") of *Every Young Man, God's Man?*

How would you talk this over with God? Write your response here as a prayer to Him.

What do you believe God wants you to do in response to this week's study?

👤👤 EVERY YOUNG MAN'S TALK
(Constructive Topics and Questions for Group Discussion)

Key Highlights from the Book for Reading Aloud and Discussing

📖 The Picking and Choosing Syndrome: Let's look at the case histories of three guys your age who are following in the footsteps of those kings from yesteryear. Brad…Jamal…Mike… 📖

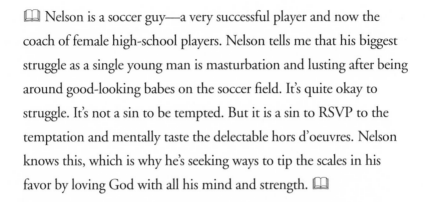 Nelson is a soccer guy—a very successful player and now the coach of female high-school players. Nelson tells me that his biggest struggle as a single young man is masturbation and lusting after being around good-looking babes on the soccer field. It's quite okay to struggle. It's not a sin to be tempted. But it is a sin to RSVP to the temptation and mentally taste the delectable hors d'oeuvres. Nelson knows this, which is why he's seeking ways to tip the scales in his favor by loving God with all his mind and strength.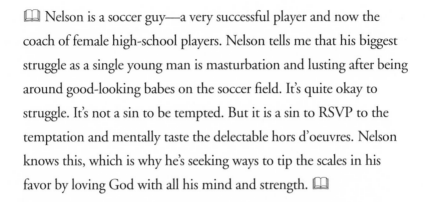

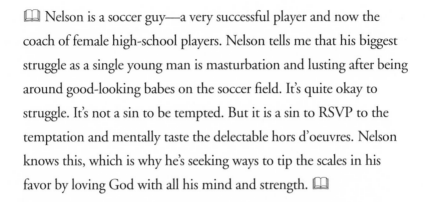 I identified with Superman and Gumby for different reasons. I think part of me wanted to be a superhero while another part of me definitely had my head in the clouds. Pretty weird combination, if you think about it. One guy was indestructible. The other was soft and bendable. The Man of Steel tried to never get bent out of shape. The green figure made of clay *always* was being handled and changed to become real to me (the viewer). Superman always prevailed over the bad guys in the end. Gumby, on the other hand, always had his heart changed by the end of an episode—in victory or defeat.

Discussion Questions

An opening question: Which parts of these chapters were most helpful or encouraging to you? Why?

A. Kenny talks about the picking and choosing syndrome. Go back and look at how Brad, Jamal, and Mike do it. Can you see yourself in any of their attitudes and actions? Tell about it.

B. What specific plan did Nelson come up with to keep himself from RSVPing to temptation? Evaluate together the strengths and weaknesses of his plan.

C. What is good about being a Gumby in your walk with God?

Section II: focus on chapters 10b
(beginning with the subhead "The Great Divide") and 11.

Note: if you're following a twelve-week track,
save the rest of this lesson for the following week.
If you're on the eight-week track…then keep going.

☑ EVERY YOUNG MAN'S CHOICE
(Questions for Personal Reflection and Examination)

📖 Then there was the time I mountain-biked down the summit of 11,053-foot-high Mammoth Mountain and felt like I was riding through someone else's yard (namely, God's). Those are the moments when I see how big and powerful He must be and how small and insignificant I am. I see David's point in real time: who am I that that He should even think of me?

When a man recognizes this God gap, there is only one way he should respond: silence. 📖

📖 Jason's revenge is a perfect illustration of baptism…. Thus Marty Wolf was baptized into the blue color because he soaked in the dye long enough for his skin to take on the character of the blue dye.

The point of baptism is that you identify with whatever you soak in.

In a similar fashion, your mind takes on the character or colors of whatever you are soaking in. When you place your life in the mirror, what's reflected back tells you what color dye your brain is soaking in. 📖

11. Read and meditate on Psalm 8, focusing on verse 4. For Kenny, God's majesty in nature brought on humility. When have you, too, felt humbled by God's total awesomeness?

12. How did the story of Jason's revenge (in the movie *Big Fat Liar*) affect you? What have you been soaking your brain in this week? during the past month?

👟 EVERY YOUNG MAN'S WALK
(Your Guide to Personal Application)

📖 God is always one up, and we're always one down. That should be enough, but we're human, so we often keep forgetting stuff like this. It helps to remember the depth of the love behind His power and His position. This makes every God's man *want* to be flexible in His hands. 📖

📖 My mental pool, which was saturated with the sexy dye of porn and mental fantasy, was slowly drained and replaced with the pure water of Christ's living words. After soaking my mind in the Word of God, I had the necessary ingredients to begin sharing my faith in Christ with others, which would eventually lead to opportunities to help thousands of men every year around the globe.

Two Kennys, two marinades, two very different directions— but one undeniable fact: the content of my mind created my character. 📖

13. Prayerfully read Isaiah 45:6-7. How is God one up on you? What is your gut-level response?

14. Check the waters in your mental swimming pool for a moment. How would you rate the purity levels?

____ A welcome sight: crystal clear and sparkling waters

____ A filter problem: dirt clinging to the bottom

____ A scrubbing challenge: ugly stains, lots of debris

____ A death trap: one stinking mess of scum and sludge

15. If you're wondering, *How do I get God's mind?* Kenny's answer is *meditation.* So choose one of the scriptures mentioned in chapter 11 of the book. Right now, spend ten minutes meditating on it. Then think: *What did I notice?*

16. Alan took his relationship with Jesus very personally. How is that different from having a disciplined devotional life?

17. What for you was the most meaningful concept or truth in chapters 10b (beginning with the subhead "The Great Divide") and 11 of *Every Young Man, God's Man?*

How would you talk this over with God? Write your response here as a prayer to Him.

What do you believe God wants you to do in response to this week's study?

EVERY YOUNG MAN'S TALK
(Constructive Topics and Questions for Group Discussion)

Key Highlights from the Book for Reading Aloud and Discussing

Young men who know better but refuse to heed God's voice create misery for themselves and for those around them. I have seen my share of guys who think they have it all figured out at eighteen or nineteen, and they frustrate the snot out of me. These guys would never think they're coming out against God, but their choices and even their questions reek of pride. Most of all, these guys isolate themselves from people of truth and plug their ears to voices of truth. It's a frustrating pattern that has been repeated for centuries among God's men. Aaron is one of the most recent examples.

📖 In the movie *Big Fat Liar,* Jason Shepherd, the main character, was not unlike a certain author who became very skillful at lying to friends and family to avoid responsibilities at school and at home. The movie's opening scenes make clear that Jason is quite good at this—he's got everyone from his principal to his parents believing his innocent and touching lies. 📖

📖 A killer statement I have never forgotten was when I heard a guy on the radio quote Samuel Smiles, a writer from the 1800s: "Sow a thought, reap an action. Sow an action, reap a habit. Sow a habit, reap a character. Sow a character, reap a destiny." Did you know that the journey of a thought has such power? If the first thing I need to know about my mind is that *I am* what I think, then the second truth I have to understand is that *I do* what I think. 📖

Discussion Questions

An opening question: Which parts of this chapter were most helpful or encouraging to you? Why?

D. Aaron thought he had it all figured out. Go back and think through his story. How did God break through Aaron's pride?

E. Have you ever been a big, fat liar? What are some of the short-term benefits of this approach to life? What are some long-term drawbacks?

F. According to Kenny, what is the first truth to know about your mind? What is the second? How well do you really know these two principles—based on your lifestyle?

G. Kenny says: "God equates studying His Word to hanging out with Him." Do you agree? What is hanging out with God like for you?

H. Together, list as many reasons you can think of for *not having enough time* to marinate yourself in God's Word. Then discuss Kenny's statement: "When a guy says to me that he doesn't have time for God's Word, he's not stating a fact, he's stating a priority."

I. Before ending your session, share your prayer requests for the coming week.

（６）

stay sharp and speak up

This week's reading assignment:

chapters 12–14 in *Every Young Man, God's Man*

Every young man needs another young man in his life to sharpen and realign him in his walk with God. To be God's young man requires placing a high value on male relationships that keep you spiritually strong. One of my favorite Scriptures says it best: "As iron sharpens iron, so one man sharpens another" (Proverbs 27:17).

Most young men I counsel overlook this important biblical principle, which is a shame.

—from chapter 12 in *Every Young Man, God's Man*

EVERY YOUNG MAN'S TRUTH
(Your Personal Journey into God's Word)

An old 1970s song says: "He ain't heavy, he's my brother." It speaks of caring for the other guy, because "his welfare is my concern," so "the load doesn't weigh me down at all."

Is it really possible to feel that way about other human beings? In the church, it's absolutely essential. As Christ's band of brothers, we are called to shoulder one another's burdens. We are to risk realness in our words. Speak the truth of our hearts. And just plain love one another. That way, we keep one another sharp for kingdom battles.

It starts by looking at Jesus, our mentor. Though He was Lord of all, He knelt to wash the feet of His brothers, declaring Himself to be their servant. Can you do it—serve the guy next to you in your small group? Really care about his problems and needs? The scriptures below will help you decide.

Carry each other's burdens, and in this way you will fulfill the law of Christ. (Galatians 6:2)

Speaking the truth in love, we will in all things grow up into him who is the Head, that is, Christ. From him the whole body, joined and held together by every supporting ligament, grows and builds itself up in love, as each part does its work....

Therefore each of you must put off falsehood and speak truthfully to his neighbor, for we are all members of one body. (Ephesians 4:15-16,25)

Above all, love each other deeply, because love covers over a multitude of sins. Offer hospitality to one another without grumbling. Each one should use whatever gift he has received to serve others, faithfully administering God's grace in its various forms. If anyone speaks, he should do it as one speaking the very words of God. If anyone serves, he should do it with the strength God provides, so that in all things God may be praised through Jesus Christ. To him be the glory and the power for ever and ever. Amen. (1 Peter 4:8-11)

1. Can you think of a time when a Christian brother really needed your help? What did you do?

2. According to Ephesians 4, why is speaking the truth an important part of our life in the body?

3. What does it mean to you that love covers a multitude of sins?

4. How would you define *hospitality* in your own words? What would it look like if the guys in your small group were offering "hospitality to one another without grumbling"?

Section I: focus on chapters 12 and 13a
(ending before the subhead "Confession Is Not for Cowards").

Note: for an eight-week study,
include Section II starting on page 72.

☑ EVERY YOUNG MAN'S CHOICE
(Questions for Personal Reflection and Examination)

📖 If you're unsharpened by the presence of another committed friend, your commitment to God won't perform. It will be duller than a steak knife that's been played with in the dirt all morning long. But a young man who's got a spiritual sharpening stone in his life—another brother headed down the same path toward God—can make the transition to the bigger issues of manhood with support, confidence, and encouragement to do the right thing.

Take Jordan for example... 📖

📖 Since I'm older and have spoken on sexual integrity issues for years, I felt at ease talking about sex to this group of students. I described how I struggled to be victorious, fought "the fever" as a younger man, and experienced the huge blessings of sexual integrity. I want younger audiences to connect with me as someone who knows *exactly* what they're going through.

That morning in Ohio, I made the following points... 📖

5. Who is your spiritual sharpening stone? How does he help you the most? Who might be a good candidate to become your sharpening stone in the future?

6. Review the points Kenny made during his talk in Ohio. Choose the one that sparks the most interest for you—and jot the reason here:

EVERY YOUNG MAN'S WALK
(Your Guide to Personal Application)

📖 Listen, the guys you think have it all together are just as whacked out as you! The discovery that is helping today's young men win their big spiritual battles is that they are learning they need better relationships with their *God-focused* peers. When I encourage young men to pursue relationships with their guy friends, I see many change their thinking about their guy connections and use them in ways that God intended. 📖

📖 Guys don't even *think* about discussing their feelings or what's churning inside with another friend. We prefer to stuff our emotions, maintain a stiff upper lip, and carry on with harboring what's really going on inside....

The result is that we're pretty bad at dealing with our emotions. Here's a quick list, and ask yourself if any of these hit your bull's-eye:

- You mask anger with sarcasm.
- You avoid serious conversations by making fun of the subject.
- You "gotta go."
- You change the scenery.
- You keep secrets.
- You avoid guilt through rationalization.
- You deflect mistakes.
- You blame others.
- You hang out with shallow people who don't "go there."
- You change the subject. 📖

7. What's the difference between a peer and a God-focused peer? How many friends of each do you have? Which relationships do you actively pursue?

8. Take up Kenny's challenge in the second quotation above and mark which two or three emotion-avoiding tactics hit your bull's-eye.

9. What for you was the most meaningful concept or truth in these chapters of *Every Young Man, God's Man?*

How would you talk this over with God? Write your response here as a prayer to Him.

What do you believe God wants you to do in response to this week's study?

EVERY YOUNG MAN'S TALK
(Constructive Topics and Questions for Group Discussion)

Key Highlights from the Book for Reading Aloud and Discussing

I know we've talked about the fairer sex a lot in *Every Young Man, God's Man,* but the number one dilemma facing God's young men today is not sexual temptation. It's isolation.

📖 I have found that young men who aren't making the transition to spiritual manhood have reached their sad state because they're connected to other guys who dull their edge to their goals as God's men. In this group of friends, they don't:

- risk getting honest about the tough stuff burning a hole in the pit of their stomachs
- watch one another's backs spiritually
- pray for one another regularly
- push one another to be in God's Word
- ask how a guy's walk with the Lord is going
- encourage one another to take bold risks for Christ
- care enough to confront behavior that doesn't square with Scripture 📖

📖 When it comes to getting honest with others about what's really going on in their lives, many young men pull the old rope-a-dope. They use spin, employ shady tactics, or just flat-out lie to deliberately lead people to thinking all is well when the reality is that they need help, advice, or even rescue. 📖

Discussion Questions

An opening question: Which parts of these chapters were most helpful or encouraging to you? Why?

A. If you agree with Kenny that isolation—not sexual temptation—is a young man's number one dilemma, how do you explain it?

B. How can another guy dull your spiritual edge? (See the seven listed don'ts.) How can he sharpen you?

C. When have you seen the old rope-a-dope in action among a group of guys? How effective was it?

D. Look again at the seven scriptures that Kenny lists to show "what God has to say about the science of being sharp." Discuss how each of these passages could apply to a twenty-first-century guy.

Section II: focus on chapters 13b
(beginning with the subhead "Confession Is Not for Cowards") and 14.

Note: if you're following a twelve-week track,
save the rest of this lesson for the following week.
If you're on the eight-week track…then keep going.

☑ EVERY YOUNG MAN'S CHOICE
(Questions for Personal Reflection and Examination)

📖 Most young men do not have the stomach for confession because it forces them to confront themselves or their actions. (Newsflash: *no one likes to do that!*) Revealing your dirty laundry is like showing the world your dirty underwear. No one wants to do that, so it's better to resort to rope-a-dope. The problem is that the only one getting roped is you! Satan loves it when a young man believes his smoke screens are working, because the longer he stays unconfessed and self-deceived, the longer he can keep inflicting losses on someone who could be living for God. 📖

📖 Most guys I counsel have not engaged the ministry of the Holy Spirit, the third person of the Trinity, and all He can do for them. Perhaps you're unaware that Jesus described His character and ministry with such words as *counselor, comforter, helper, spirit of truth,* and *guide.* The Holy Spirit is ready and willing to speak the right direction in your mind. All you have to do is let Him do this, and when that happens, He will guide you through every temptation and help you avoid many of the traps others fall into. 📖

10. In silence, with a heart open to God, reflect:

Do I have a stomach for confession?

Have I been rope-a-doping lately?

How unconfessed am I at the moment?

11. Would you like to engage the ministry of the Holy Spirit today? Well, just let Him. Jot your request to the Holy Spirit here:

📖 EVERY YOUNG MAN'S WALK
(Your Guide to Personal Application)

📖 I look at confession as giving Satan a bloody nose, and that's what happens when you punch back with God's truth.

If you think I'm off base on this, just listen to how strongly God encourages His people to practice the discipline of confession with Him and others, then make a note of the consequences. 📖

📖 For God's young man, trusting that the Holy Spirit will be there to guide you and counsel you is kind of like taking that first run down the bunny slope. It's a risk because you're practically guaranteed to fall. But one thing I've learned about being God's young man is that when you risk changing for Him, the change always takes you to the next level. Spiritually speaking, you'll go from the bunny slopes to carving some serious powder in the back bowls. 📖

12. You can rely on God's Word and give Satan a bloody nose! Meditate on the scriptures below and jot the consequences of practicing—or *not* practicing—the discipline of confession.

Psalm 51:6

Proverbs 28:13

James 5:16

1 John 1:8-9

13. When you face temptation or tough times, does it feel risky to switch from willpower to relying on the Holy Spirit? Why? What can make this kind of reliance more of a habit in a guy's life?

14. Go to the prayer that appears toward the end of chapter 14. Consider whether you'd like to make those words your own. If so, spend a few moments offering them to the Holy Spirit with a sincere heart.

15. What for you was the most meaningful concept or truth in these chapter readings from *Every Young Man, God's Man?*

How would you talk this over with God? Write your response here as a prayer to Him.

What do you believe God wants you to do in response to this week's study?

EVERY YOUNG MAN'S TALK
(Constructive Topics and Questions for Group Discussion)

Key Highlights from the Book for Reading Aloud and Discussing

Rich approached me and asked to speak in private. When we got out of earshot of the other guys, he put it straight to me: "I really wonder what's in it for me if I come clean about masturbation and surfing adult Web sites with my college group. Won't people be angry with me since I've got this junk in my life and I'm supposed to be a leader? Can't I just come clean with you and that's it?"

"Do you want victory?" I replied.

"Absolutely," he said.

"Then here's what you say to your group…" 📖

📖 Practice under pressure over time creates confidence. 📖

📖 God has spelled out exactly how He wants to use the Holy Spirit in your life and how you, as God's young man, need to start working with Him. Like any relationship, the first step is to learn more about Him so that you can partner more closely. And what a great partner He is! The Holy Spirit can… 📖

Discussion Questions

An opening question: Which parts of this chapter were most helpful or encouraging to you? Why?

E. Do you agree that Rich needed to bring things out into the open with his guys' small group? If you were him, how nervous would you be at the moment of truth?

F. Kenny lists ten things the Holy Spirit can do. Go through them, one by one, in your group. Comment on how these truths can be encouraging to guys like you. Be as specific and practical as possible.

G. One of Kenny's favorite sayings is: "Practice under pressure over time creates confidence." What's your opinion about it? How does it apply to the challenge of learning to depend on the Holy Spirit?

H. Have everyone look at the prayer to the Holy Sprit found at the end of chapter 14. Ask one another: "Who prayed this prayer when you were filling in your workbook before the group time?" Spend some time sharing about who has prayed—and who would *like* to pray— these words for themselves.

power, pressure, and progress

I kept pedaling and pedaling, and five and a half hours later I crossed the finish line, crying for my mama. I finished a respectable sixty-first, which was in the middle of the pack. But more important, I learned a huge lesson. All I had to do was get on the bike, strengthen my legs, and let them carry me to the end.

Mountain biking is all about power and performance, and if you've got no power, you've got no performance....

Power is a good thing, and prayer is the outlet that God has chosen to connect you to His vast reservoir of power.

—from chapter 15 in *Every Young Man, God's Man*

EVERY YOUNG MAN'S TRUTH
(Your Personal Journey into God's Word)

Pressure and prayer. They really are related, as you'll see in this session. Logically, it makes sense: when trouble hits, you go to God.

Sadly, many of us make a pit stop first. We first try to engineer our way out. We throw all our own power at the problem. Then, if things don't work out, we come before God with hat in hand.

Is it just a sign of laziness? "Why are you sleeping?" Jesus asked His friends when they should have been praying. Is He asking you the same tough question?

Be still, and know that I am God. (Psalm 46:10)

Jesus went out as usual to the Mount of Olives, and his disciples followed him. On reaching the place, he said to them, "Pray that you will not fall into temptation." He withdrew about a stone's throw beyond them, knelt down and prayed, "Father, if you are willing, take this cup from me; yet not my will, but yours be done." An angel from heaven appeared to him and strengthened him. And being in anguish, he prayed more earnestly, and his sweat was like drops of blood falling to the ground.

When he rose from prayer and went back to the disciples, he found them asleep, exhausted from sorrow. "Why are you sleeping?" he asked them. "Get up and pray so that you will not fall into temptation." (Luke 22:39-46)

Do not throw away your confidence; it will be richly rewarded. You need to persevere so that when you have done the will of God, you will receive what he has promised. For in just a very little while,

"He who is coming will come and will not delay.
But my righteous one will live by faith.
And if he shrinks back,
I will not be pleased with him."

But we are not of those who shrink back and are destroyed, but of those who believe and are saved. (Hebrews 10:35-39)

1. In a typical day, when are you still before God?

2. According to Jesus, how does prayer relate to our temptation battles?

3. How does God view your willingness to persevere in tough times? Why?

4. How would you like to improve your prayer life? What first step could you take today?

Section I: focus on chapter 15. Note: for an eight-week
study, include Section II starting on page 86.

☑ EVERY YOUNG MAN'S CHOICE
(Questions for Personal Reflection and Examination)

📖 We cannot fathom how many lives are affected every day by
Google. Yet all of that astonishing power cannot come close to the
storehouse of personal spiritual power available to you as God's
young servant, which is made possible through the power of
prayer.... There is a living spiritual engine within you that can
search the mind of God for... 📖

📖 Josh's scenario is typical of most young men when it comes to
prayer: it took a crisis situation before it even dawned on him to talk
to God in prayer. Let's put it this way: Josh was certainly mindful of
God when he needed something or when he was in a setting that
called for prayer, like during chapel or when his Bible study was fin-
ishing up. He realizes that his dialogue with God is shallow and self-
ish most of the time (like today), but he can't seem to work in more
conversations with God.

Do you ever wonder what the Creator thinks when He views this
kind of prayer life? Isaiah heard it loud and clear: "And so the Lord
says, 'These people say they are mine. They honor me with their lips,
but their hearts are far from me'" (Isaiah 29:13, NLT). 📖

5. Think about the Google-smashing power of God within you as you
   prayerfully read Ephesians 3:20. Then go over Kenny's list of ten

needs that God's power can meet. Which of these needs are pressuring you right now?

6. How is your prayer life like or unlike Josh's?

7. Kenny says, *"Prayer is the power that fuels the performance of your faith."* What comment, question, or personal experience does this bring to your mind?

🥾 EVERY YOUNG MAN'S WALK
(Your Guide to Personal Application)

📖 God is waiting for you to access His awesome strength. Everything is just a prayer away. If you're clueless to the personal benefits of prayer, or in too much of a hurry to slow down and get into the practice of prayer, here's what you need to know: your network card was installed in you at salvation, and talking to God is done wirelessly. So what are you waiting for? 📖

📖 Prayer, for you, is a secret power, an adventure in trusting the living God. When a young man recognizes this privilege, he moves beyond the task of prayer to the treasure of being present with God. As Scripture says, "A single day in your courts is better than a thousand anywhere else!" (Psalm 84:10, NLT) 📖

8. Imagine God *waiting* for you to connect with Him in prayer. Are you mostly…

____ "clueless to the personal benefits of prayer"?

____ "in too much of a hurry to slow down and get into the practice of prayer"?

____ ready to slow down for God in a prayer relationship?

9. How can Kenny call *being present with God* a treasure? What is this treasure's value to you, based on your prayer practices?

10. Rewrite Psalm 84:10 here in your own words.

11. What for you was the most meaningful concept or truth in chapter 15 of *Every Young Man, God's Man?*

How would you talk this over with God? Write your response here as a prayer to Him.

What do you believe God wants you to do in response to this week's study?

Every Young Man's Talk
(Constructive Topics and Questions for Group Discussion)

Key Highlights from the Book for Reading Aloud and Discussing

Josh reviewed how his day was going so far. *Let's see. First the test—no better than a B-minus or C for sure. Then my parents—I'll have to fake like I'm doing good in school. I'll have to work to pay for those*

Christmas presents—and that Cindy—oh, mama. Not good. What next? How did I get here? He pocketed his cell phone, took a huge breath, and cupped his face in his hands. Lord, what do I do? 📖

📖 For Jesus, quick connection and quality relationship was an oxymoron—two totally contradictory ideas that don't go together. The message to Martha was simple: *You can't connect with Me on the fly!* He wouldn't cheat Martha's sister, Mary, out of their time together by cutting it short. But I know plenty of young men who have cut Jesus short on prayer because they simply don't know how to slow down, relax, and talk with their Savior about stuff. 📖

📖 Trying to manage your life without praying is like trying to ride a bike with flat tires. It can be done, but life is sure going to be tiring, laborious, and no fun. You certainly can't enjoy the ride or feel the wind in your face. Only a total dork would choose to do that, but that is exactly what you are choosing to do if you neglect the power of prayer. 📖

Discussion Questions

An opening question: Which parts of these chapters were most helpful or encouraging to you? Why?

A. Ever had a day like Josh's? How much do you pray on those kinds of days? on normal days? on good days?

B. Ask one of the guys to read aloud the story of Mary and Martha in Luke 10:38-42. How deeply has Jesus's message to these women—that *you can't connect with Me on the fly*—sunk into your own heart?

C. Who in your group will admit to living like a dork (according to Kenny's definition)? What could help you repair those flat tires on your prayer bike?

D. A key point in this study session is that Jesus wants to be with you. How does this make you feel?

Section II: focus on chapter 16.

Note: if you're following a twelve-week track,
save the rest of this lesson for the following week.
If you're on the eight-week track…then keep going.

☑ EVERY YOUNG MAN'S CHOICE
(Questions for Personal Reflection and Examination)

📖 After Miss Trench Coat's unexpected appearance, however, I felt like Daniel in a pagan palace asked to swallow food offered to idols. I could not stomach this, nor could I participate in it. But what else could I do? It was just me against a tidal wave of testosterone. 📖

📖 God taught me a powerful lesson that day: pressure is a good thing, because it never leaves you where it finds you. What I mean is that there were only two directions I could have taken. I could have joined in the fun and compromised. Or I could make the best stand under the circumstances and fight with the tools God gave me. In the end, I faced ninety minutes of pressure—from the announcement during dinner to the striptease act, but I received a clear view of God's awesome power. 📖

12. If you had been Kenny in the Miss Trench Coat crisis, what do you think you would have done?

13. What have you learned about pressure so far in your life? How did you learn these things?

14. Kenny says you need God's overpowering strength with you to equalize the pressure being put on you by the world, the dark side, and the devil. Look at the fifteen pressures he lists on page 206. Think:

Which of these are my own pressures and struggles?

What pressures would I add to this list?

What scriptures in this session could help me apply an equalizer?

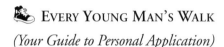 EVERY YOUNG MAN'S WALK
(Your Guide to Personal Application)

   📖 When I realized that I led a parade of none, I stomped up
to my room on the second floor, my blood boiling and my mind
spinning. Part of me wished that I was still on the other side so I
wouldn't have this intense battle raging inside. The other part of me
said, *Fight!* 📖

   📖 When similar situations come your way, think of how God wants
to use this pressure to make you a new man. Most young men have a
one-sided view of pressure, temptation, and trials—a negative one.
But that's how the world, the dark side, and Satan want you to see it.
God wants you to see it His way. 📖

15. When have you felt like Kenny as he stomped back to his room?
    What do you usually do when you are feeling yanked between the
    other side and the call to fight?

16. What positive results did Kenny experience because of his choices about Miss Trench Coat? What does this tell you about the role of pressure in a guy's life?

17. What for you was the most meaningful concept or truth in chapter 16 of *Every Young Man, God's Man?*

How would you talk this over with God? Write your response here as a prayer to Him.

What do you believe God wants you to do in response to this week's study?

EVERY YOUNG MAN'S TALK

(Constructive Topics and Questions for Group Discussion)

Key Highlights from the Book for Reading Aloud and Discussing

📖 Suddenly, a searing thought landed like a grenade in a foxhole: *Pray Miss Trench Coat out of there.* 📖

📖 God's plan to make you a man doesn't include a provision to remove you from pressure. In fact, He's most likely to *throw* you into pressure-packed situations, because He knows that will increase your faith and grow your character in Christ. More often than not, you'll have to choose God and trust Him with the results. God tests you because you're still growing up. 📖

📖 You'll likely experience ups and downs and the occasional face plant, but that's okay because you aren't perfect (nor am I). Only one man scored a perfect ten on earth, and He's not you! So just chill out and cut yourself some slack, because God certainly does. Listen to His encouraging voice speak to your journey…Proverbs 24:16… Philippians 2:12-13…Philippians 1:6…Proverbs 4:18. 📖

Discussion Questions

An opening question: Which parts of this chapter were most helpful or encouraging to you? Why?

E. Kenny prayed Miss Trench Coat out of the room. Talk about the power of prayer for a few minutes. Do you have any personal stories to share about this?

F. Name some things that grow stronger under pressure. Then read 2 Corinthians 12:9-10 and discuss how God's young man can grow stronger under pressure.

G. When have you done a face plant under pressure in the past? How could these scriptures help at a time like that?

Proverbs 24:16

Philippians 2:12-13

Philippians 1:6

Proverbs 4:18

H. Kenny tells us that perseverance under pressure pleases God. Then he lists nine ways to equalize that pressure. Look at each item on his list and tell whether you have ever tried it yourself. What happened?

I. English evangelist Charles H. Spurgeon said: "I owe more to the fire and hammer and file than anything else in my Lord's work-shop." If Spurgeon were to visit your group right now, would you give him a high-five for this statement? Why or why not?

plan the victory, honor the sacrifice

This week's reading assignment:

chapters 17–18 in *Every Young Man, God's Man*

If you're really serious about your relationship to God, then you'll agree that wise planning reduces temptation. When you deal with issues before *you're tempted, you enter the battle with a plan versus just showing up clueless about what happens next. When you execute a plan like this, you're counting the cost of what it takes to build a solid spiritual life.*

—from chapter 17 in *Every Young Man, God's Man*

EVERY YOUNG MAN'S TRUTH
(Your Personal Journey into God's Word)

First you plan. Then you realize the limits of your plan. Which brings you to the unlimited effectiveness of the Cross. That's what this session is all about: your call to plan for your battles with the dark side and your need to rely, ultimately, on the sacrifice of Christ for your victories.

But really, how important is the Cross to you? Do you realize that without it you would have no hope of eternal life? Do you understand that by the Cross, you were forgiven and made a child of God? If you know these things, how could you respond with anything but gratitude in your daily life? It boils down to this: honor the sacrifice!

> Suppose one of you wants to build a tower. Will he not first sit down and estimate the cost to see if he has enough money to complete it? For if he lays the foundation and is not able to finish it, everyone who sees it will ridicule him, saying, "This fellow began to build and was not able to finish." (Luke 14:28-30)

> He grew up before him like a tender shoot,
>   and like a root out of dry ground.
> He had no beauty or majesty to attract us
>   to him,
>   nothing in his appearance that we should
>   desire him.
> He was despised and rejected by men,
>   a man of sorrows, and familiar with suffering.
> Like one from whom men hide their faces
>   he was despised, and we esteemed him not.
> Surely he took up our infirmities
>   and carried our sorrows,
> yet we considered him stricken by God,
>   smitten by him, and afflicted.
> But he was pierced for our transgressions,
>   he was crushed for our iniquities;
> the punishment that brought us peace was
>   upon him,
>   and by his wounds we are healed.

We all, like sheep, have gone astray,
>> each of us has turned to his own way;
and the LORD has laid on him
>> the iniquity of us all.
He was oppressed and afflicted,
>> yet he did not open his mouth;
he was led like a lamb to the slaughter,
>> and as a sheep before her shearers is silent,
>> so he did not open his mouth.
>> (Isaiah 53:2-7)

And he died for all, that those who live should no longer live for themselves but for him who died for them and was raised again. (2 Corinthians 5:15)

1. When have you left a job unfinished due to poor planning? What did you learn?

2. Some people plan how they will get to heaven. Is it possible to punch your own ticket to the Pearly Gates? Which Scripture truths above help you answer?

3. Carefully read through the Isaiah passage above. How does the idea of substitution come through to you?

4. The Cross is about *dying,* but what does it have to do with *living?*

☑ EVERY YOUNG MAN'S CHOICE
(Questions for Personal Reflection and Examination)

📖 As God's young man, you, too, must have a plan for the key battles in your future. In these circumstances, it helps to think like General Patton for a second. The following questions are designed to help facilitate your planning process… 📖

📖 Jesus knew how to get a man's attention—and I'm just glad He didn't mention other parts of the male anatomy! What He was saying in blunt language was this:

- Sin is the enemy.
- Cut sin off at the source.
- Keep God and eternity in mind as you make choices.
- Know your weaknesses so that you can cut them out effectively. 📖

5. Think about your plans for righteous living. Go back to the book's list of questions to help facilitate the planning process (under the subhead "Cutting Off and Starving Sin"). Then spend several minutes answering these questions for your own life.

6. Read Mark 9:43-48. How serious is our sin in God's eyes?

7. Kenny says that for every excuse young men may give, there is a bloodstained cross staring back at them. What emotional power does that cross have in your life?

EVERY YOUNG MAN'S WALK
(Your Guide to Personal Application)

  Predetermined boundaries may involve cutting off and starving sin in the following ways:

- carving sexy R-rated films out of your cinematic repertoire
- deciding that the bar scene or drinking parties will not be the place where you connect with friends
- refusing to keep sexual secrets that put distance between you and God
- accepting sexual accountability
- inviting people you spiritually respect to ask you the tough questions
- committing to not mentally undressing any woman
- getting software that allows someone to see where you have been on the Net
- committing in writing with a girl you're dating the dos and don'ts of the physical relationship.

  Jesus stood in the observation post at one time. He was our forward observer who saw the potential of sin to overwhelm and destroy your life. Then He called for fire directly on His position, saying, in a sense, "Put it all on Me!" And that's when hell and death and sin fell upon Him. Friends protested. "Never, Lord!" said Peter, but Jesus refused to back off. He turned toward His Father and said, "I want your will, not mine" (Luke 22:42, NLT).

How do you honor that kind of sacrifice? By making it a part of your life.

8. Which of the cut-off-and-starve activities hit closest to home?

9. How do you honor the Cross in your life? What qualities are there, in your words and actions, that demonstrate your respect?

10. In quietness, review what you have written and learned in this week's study. If further thoughts or prayer requests come to your mind and heart, you may want to write them here.

11. What for you was the most meaningful concept or truth in this week's study?

How would you talk this over with God? Write your response here as a prayer to Him.

What do you believe God wants you to do in response to this week's study?

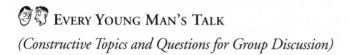 EVERY YOUNG MAN'S TALK
(Constructive Topics and Questions for Group Discussion)

Key Highlights from the Book for Reading Aloud and Discussing

📖 One of the reasons so many young men suffer defeat regularly in spiritual warfare is that they fail to engage the Enemy or take a proactive approach to battle. They just show up and expect that's enough to conquer direct attacks against their faith. If Patton thought like that, we might all be speaking German today. 📖

📖 The things that a guy tends to resist—limits, godly boundaries, and rules—are the very things you need to become the man God wants you to be. The dark side, the popular culture, and the devil will attempt to convince you that these commitments are old school and take away your independence. In my experience, most young guys who believe this become slaves to the very attitudes and actions they were told represented freedom. 📖

📖 Charles H. Spurgeon so aptly said, "A dying Savior is the death of sin." 📖

Discussion Questions

An opening question: Which parts of these chapters were most helpful or encouraging to you? Why?

A. What does it mean to be proactive in spiritual warfare?

B. Why do we tend to resist limits, boundaries, and rules? How does this show up in your life?

C. What did Spurgeon mean by his statement about a dying Savior? Answer by explaining your own theology of the Cross.

D. Kenny challenges us to never, ever, ever forget the price that Christ paid for our sin. Do you believe you could ever forget? Why?

E. Since this is your last session together in this study, spend some time talking about what you've learned and how you've changed. Then share prayer requests about your desires for further growth as God's young men.

don't keep it to yourself

If you've just completed the *Every Young Man, God's Man Workbook* on your own, and you found it to be a helpful and valuable experience, we encourage you to consider organizing a group of your peers and helping lead them through the book and workbook together.

You'll find more information about starting such a group in the section titled "Questions You May Have About This Workbook."

about the authors

STEPHEN ARTERBURN is coauthor of the best-selling Every Man series. He is founder and chairman of New Life Clinics, host of the daily "New Life Live!" national radio program, creator of the Women of Faith Conferences, a nationally known speaker and licensed minister, and the author of more than forty books. He lives with his family in Laguna Beach, California.

KENNY LUCK is president and founder of Every Man Ministries and co-author of the best-selling *Every Man, God's Man* and its companion work-book. He is the men's minister and a member of the teaching staff of Saddleback Valley Community Church in Lake Forest, California. He and his wife, Chrissy, have three children and reside in Rancho Santa Margarita, California.

MIKE YORKEY is the author, coauthor, or general editor of more than thirty books, including all the books in the Every Man series. He and his wife, Nicole, are the parents of two college-age children and live in Encinitas, California.

the best-selling every man series—
for men in hot pursuit
of God's best in every area of life

Go beyond easy answers and glib treatments to discover powerful, practical guidance that makes a difference in men's lives—and in their relationships with God, the women in their lives, their friends, and the world.

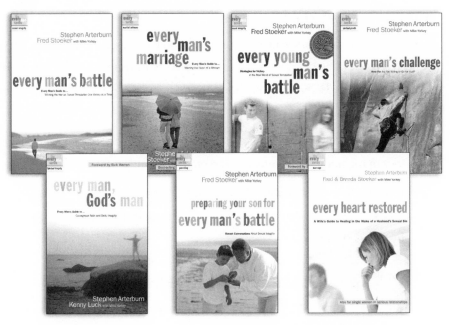

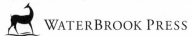

WATERBROOK PRESS

every man's battle workshops

from New Life Ministries

New Life Ministries receives hundreds of calls every month from Christian men who are struggling to stay pure in the midst of daily challenges to their sexual integrity and from pastors who are looking for guidance in how to keep fragile marriages from falling apart all around them.

As part of our commitment to equip individuals to win these battles, New Life Ministries has developed biblically based workshops directly geared to answer these needs. These workshops are held several times per year around the country.

- Our workshops **for men** are structured to equip men with the tools necessary to maintain sexual integrity and enjoy healthy, productive relationships.

- Our workshops **for church leaders** are targeted to help pastors and men's ministry leaders develop programs to help families being attacked by this destructive addiction.

Some comments from previous workshop attendees:

"An awesome, life-changing experience. Awesome teaching, teacher, content and program." —DAVE

"God has truly worked a great work in me since the EMB workshop. I am fully confident that with God's help, I will be restored in my ministry position. Thank you for your concern. I realize that this is a battle, but I now have the weapons of warfare as mentioned in Ephesians 6:10, and I am using them to gain victory!" —KEN

"It's great to have a workshop you can confidently recommend to anyone without hesitation, knowing that it is truly life changing. Your labors are not in vain!" —DR. BRAD STENBERG, Pasadena, CA

If sexual temptation is threatening your marriage or your church, please call **1-800-NEW-LIFE** to speak with one of our specialists.

start a bible study
and connect with others
who want to be God's man.

Every Man Bible Studies are designed to help you discover, own, and build on convictions grounded in God's word. Available now in bookstores.

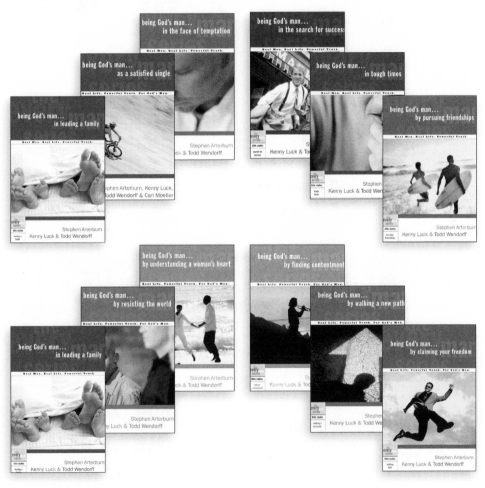

WATERBROOK
PRESS

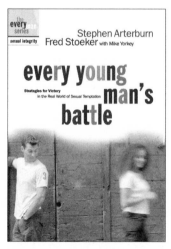